INTERMITTENT FASTING FOR WOMEN

Mary Jackson

©2019 Blanco Publishing

ISBN: 978-1-099-55953-2

INTRODUCTION

For ladies who are keen on weight loss, intermittent fasting may appear to be an extraordinary decision, yet numerous individuals need to know, should ladies quick? Is intermittent fasting successful for ladies? There have been a couple of critical examinations about intermittent fasting, which can reveal some insight into this fascinating new dietary trend.

Intermittent fasting is otherwise called exchange day fasting, although there are absolutely a few minor departures from this eating routine. The American Journal of Clinical Nutrition played out an investigation as of late that enlisted 16 hefty people on a 10-week program. On the fasting days, participants consumed food to 25% of their assessed vitality needs. The remainder of the time, they got dietary advising, however, were not given a specific rule to pursue amid this time.

True to form, the participants shed pounds because of this investigation; however, what analysts indeed discovered intriguing were some specific changes. The subjects were all still hefty after only ten weeks, yet they had appeared in cholesterol, LDL-cholesterol, triglycerides, and systolic circulatory strain. What made this an intriguing find was that the vast majority need to lose more weight than these examination participants before observing similar changes. It was a captivating discover which has urged an extraordinary number of individuals to take a stab at fasting.

Discontinuous fasting for ladies has some beneficial impacts. What makes it particularly significant for ladies who are attempting to get thinner is that ladies have a lot greater large extent in their bodies. When endeavoring to get in shape, the body fundamentally consumes carbohydrate stores with the first 6 hours and after that begins to consume fat. Ladies who are following a healthy eating regimen and exercise plan might battle with stubborn fat, yet fasting is a practical answer for this.

Discontinuous Fasting For Women Over 50

Our bodies and our digestion changes when we hit menopause. One of the most significant changes that ladies more than 50 experience is that they have slower digestion, and they begin to put on weight. Fasting might be a suitable method to switch and counteract this weight gain, however. Studies have demonstrated that this fasting design manages hunger, and individuals who tail it consistently don't encounter similar longings that others do. In case you're more than 50 and endeavoring to conform to your slower digestion, intermittent fasting can assist you with avoiding eating a lot every day.

When you achieve 50, your body likewise begins to build up some unending infections like elevated cholesterol and hypertension. Discontinuous fasting has been appeared to diminish both cholesterol and circulatory strain, even without a lot of weight loss. If you've begun to see your numbers ascending at the specialist's office every year, you might most likely carry them down with fasting, even without losing much weight.

Intermittent fasting may not be an extraordinary thought for each lady. Anybody with a specific health condition or who will, in general, be hypoglycemic ought to counsel with a specialist. This new dietary trend has particular advantages for ladies who usually store progressively fat in their bodies and may experience difficulty disposing of these fat stores.

CHAPTER ONE

Intermittent Fasting for Women

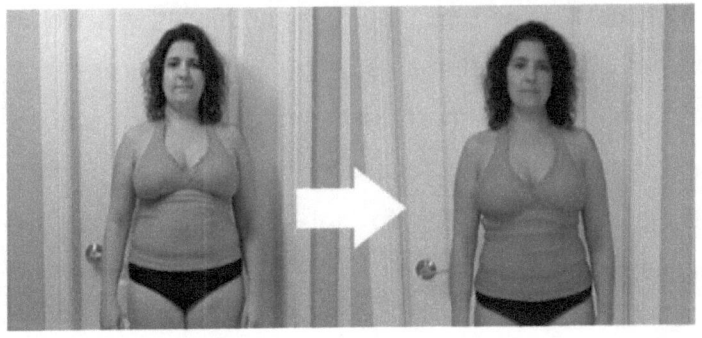

Intermittent fasting, otherwise called IF, has turned into a common technique for getting lean and shedding pounds. It's likewise said to support vitality levels, increment inspiration and stamina, and improve mental capacity. Those advantages don't sound excessively ratty, isn't that right?

While intermittent fasting seems to offer some encouraging advantages, it may not be for everybody — mainly relying upon whether you're male or female. Furthermore, as it stands now, there's more research being done on intermittent fasting for rodents than for people.

It appears that whether intermittent fasting will work for you boils down to human science. While shorter times of fasting are, for the most part, thought to be alright for a great many people, a portion of the all-encompassing fasting times related to intermittent fasting aren't suggested for ladies.

Before we dive into the subtleties, how about we take a gander at what intermittent fasting is, how it works, and the upsides and downsides of this eating pattern for ladies.

What is Intermittent Fasting and How Does it Work?

Intermittent fasting may sound somewhat specialized. However, you've most likely done it before without acknowledging it. To start with, it knows the difference between the fasted state and sustained state.

The Fasted State versus Sustained State

When you eat like clockwork, that is no joke "sustained" state, which is the point at which your body is caught up with processing, retaining, and acclimatizing the supplements from your meals. Quickened fat consuming isn't the #1 need here. The more significant part of us stays in the fed state amid the day, besides when we're dozing.

The motivation behind why intermittent fasting can give certain advantages to weight reduction is because it enables your body to enter the fasted state, which is the point at which your muscle to fat ratio's consuming can indeed quicken.

How Intermittent Fasting Works

Intermittent fasting implies you go a timeframe without eating, more often than not between 12 to 48 hours. This period is known as your fasting window, amid which time you devour fluids, for example, water, natural tea, or juices.

A few specialists prescribe drinking low-calorie green vegetable squeezes and taking enhancements while fasting to help keep nutrient and mineral admission reliable, while others accept just water ought to be expended. In the same way as other themes in the wellbeing domain, the rules around intermittent fasting are emotional, contingent upon who you inquire.

If you are quick for under 24 hours, you'll likewise have an eating window. This is the time assigned for meals before you start your shift. For a great many people rehearsing intermittent fasting, their eating window is between six to 12 hours. The most widely recognized fasting times are 12,14,16 and 18 hours.

For instance, if you somehow managed to complete a 12-hour quick, your eating window would be 12 hours. You could begin your eating window at 7 am and end at 7 pm. You would break the fast the following day at 7 am.

Albeit a portion of the intermittent fasting strategies online appear to be more extraordinary than others (some can last upwards of 48 hours), the excellence of intermittent fasting is that you get the opportunity to pick and try different things with to what extent you quick. This not just enables you to decide how intermittent fasting can fit in inside your way of life, however, to find the fasting sweet recognize that encourages you to feel best physically.

Upsides and downsides of Intermittent Fasting for Women (And Why it very well may Be Tricky)

A portion of the advantages of intermittent fasting may include:

- Economic weight reduction
- An expansion in slender bulk
- More vitality
- An extension in cell stress reaction
- A decrease in oxidative pressure and aggravation
- Improvement around insulin affectability in overweight ladies
- Expanded generation of neurotrophic development factor (which could help subjective capacity)

Presently, here's the precarious part. Albeit intermittent fasting may have its advantages, ladies are generally delicate to indications of starvation, so intermittent fasting for ladies is an entire diverse brute.

At the point when the female body detects it's going towards starvation, it will build the generation of the appetite hormones, ghrelin, and leptin, which signal the body that you're eager and need to eat (2). Moreover, if there's insufficient nourishment for you to endure, your body will close down the framework that would enable you to make another human. This is the body's standard method for ensuring a potential pregnancy, regardless of whether you're not pregnant or endeavoring to consider.

It isn't so much that you're deliberately forcing starvation upon yourself — however, your body doesn't realize that. It doesn't understand the difference between actual starvation and intermittent fasting, which is the reason it defaults to this defensive instrument.

Hence, a portion of the cons because of uneven hormonal characters expedited by intermittent fasting may likewise prompt:

- Irregular periods (or complete loss of period)
- Metabolic pressure
- Contracting of the ovaries
- Tension

- Richness issues
- Trouble resting

Since the majority of your hormones are so profoundly interconnected, when one hormone is startled, the rest are likewise contrarily affected. It resembles a domino impact. As the "detachments" that control almost every capacity in your body — from vitality generation to assimilation, digestion, and circulatory strain — you would prefer not to disturb their good mood.

With these disadvantages, you might ponder: would you be able to (and would regardless you need to) practice intermittent fasting as a female? If you adopt a progressively loosened up strategy, the appropriate response is yes. At the point when done inside a briefer period, intermittent fasting may, in any case, help you achieve your weight reduction objectives and give different advantages recently referenced, without destroying your hormones.

The Best Intermittent Fasting Methods for Women

Anyway, what precisely is an unexpected way to deal with intermittent fasting? Once more, since there's little research done on intermittent fasting, we're managing somewhat of a dark area. The suppositions additionally will in general shift contingent upon which site you visit or which wellbeing master you inquire. From what we've discovered, the general rules to brief intermittent fasting for ladies are:

- Do not quick for longer than 24 hours on end

- Ideally quick for 12 to 16 hours.

- Do not quick on continuous days amid your initial half a month of fasting (for example, when you complete a 16-hour fast, do it three days seven days rather than seven)

- Drink a lot of liquids (bone stock, homegrown tea, water) amid your quick

- Only do light exercise on fasting days, for example, yoga, strolling, running, and delicate extending

Alternatives for Intermittent Fasting

There are a few unique intermittent fasting techniques talked about on the web. Here are a couple of the most prominent ones.

Crescendo Method

The Crescendo Method is a standout amongst the ideal approaches to slide into intermittent fasting without stunning your body or irritating your hormones. It doesn't expect you to be quick consistently, just a couple of days of the week, divided evenly — for instance, Monday, Wednesday and Friday.

- Fasting Window: 12-16 hours
- Eating Window: 8-12 hours
- Alright for Women: Yes
- 16/8 Method

The 16/8 technique, at times called the "lean gains strategy," is another short intermittent fasting schedule that is utilized explicitly to target muscle versus fat and improve fit bulk (a.k.a. your additions!).

- Fasting Window: 16 hours
- Eating Window: 8 hours
- Ok for Women: Yes
- 24 Hour Protocol (a.k.a. "Eat-Stop-Eat")

The 24-hour convention, otherwise called "eat-stop-eat" expects you to complete a 24-hour quick, on more than one occasion per week. You can pick the time you begin fasting. A few people want to quick from 8 pm to 8 pm the next day or start their quick after breakfast.

- **Fasting Window:** 24 hours

- **Eating Window:** 0

- **Alright for Women:** Yes, when completed a limit of 2 times each week.

The 5:2 Diet

The 5:2 eating regimen, otherwise called the "Quick Diet," includes confining calories two days seven days to 500 calories for each day (with two 250 calorie meals), while eating typically for the other five days. For instance, you may eat the majority of your regular meals Saturday through Wednesday, and eat 500 calories for each day on Thursdays and Fridays. There is anything but a large measure of research to back up this eating routine since it doesn't confine nourishment on the fasting days, it might likewise be a compelling method to slide into fasting without stunning your framework. The Fast Diet is viewed as safe for people.

Fasting Window: No fasting window, just calorie confinement to 500 calories for each day for two fasting days of the week

Eating Window: Assume regular caloric admission five days of the week

Ok for Women: Generally thought to be ok for ladies, however, contemplates are missing on this eating regimen

Strategy	Eating Window	Fasting Window	Safe for Women?
Crescendo Fasting	8-12 hours	12-16 hours	Yes
16/8 Method	8	16	Yes

The 5:2 Diet   Regular meals five days out of each week 500 calories for each day for two days of the week generally yes

When Should You Avoid Intermittent Fasting?

Intermittent fasting is certifiably not a solid match for everybody. You shouldn't consider intermittent fasting on the off chance that you are:

- Pregnant
- Nursing
- Under perpetual pressure
- Have a history of dietary issues
- Experience issues dozing

Also, intermittent fasting is intended to supplement a sound eating regimen and way of life — not go about as an approach to cure five days of eating healthfully bankrupt sustenances, for example, refined sugar, handled nourishments and quick nourishment.

Last Thoughts on Intermittent Fasting for Women

Intermittent fasting may work incredibly well for specific individuals, and awfully for other people. In particular, if you do choose out intermittent fasting an attempt, make sure to tune in to your body's input. Slipping into intermittent fasting by beginning with shorter fasting windows can help with initial symptoms of yearning and uneasiness.

10 Common Intermittent Fasting Myths

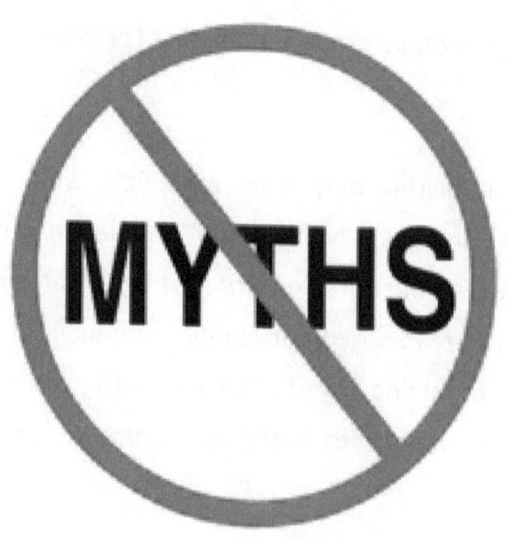

Intermittent fasting is the act of abandoning nourishment for longer timeframes than you are utilized to. You may likewise now and again hear it alluded to as time-limited eating. There are numerous extraordinary advantages of limiting the time window wherein you expend your calories for the afternoon. Anyway, many misguided judgments still exist. The motivation behind this part is to dissipate the most common fasting myths so you can feel increasingly significant utilizing this fantastic system into your daily life.

That being stated, not every person can deal with a 16 hour quick consistently. A few people find that they have a sweet spot wherein they feel and play out their best. Intermittent fasting techniques will likewise be quickly sketched out so you can have a superior thought of how to execute them into your life.

What Qualifies as Intermittent Fasting

As was referenced as of now, fasting is not expending calories for a timeframe. When you are sleeping during the evening, you are fasting. It has turned out to be well known in the wellbeing and execution network to take this window and extend it for the duration of the morning to exploit higher vitality levels, mental clarity, and improved capacity to consume fat.

Another way intermittent fasting is alluded to is by the name time-limited eating. This is because you are just making a little window of time amid the day in which you are devouring sustenance.

There are various methods for approaching fasting, including straightforward, cycle, reliable, and warrior fasting windows that happen daily and are presented underneath. One of the common intermittent fasting myths is that it must be done each day; this isn't the situation notwithstanding. Indeed, even merely performing one 24-hour quick every week has its advantages. Individuals likewise have achievement fasting each other day or two times per week.

Why Fasting Can be Beneficial

Not eating for a timeframe can be extremely helpful for the body. Intermittent fasting boosts the resistant framework, animates the tidy up and reusing of old harmed cells, improves DNA fix, improves insulin sensitivity, and ensures the body against various sicknesses.

Moreover, if you are somebody who experiences ceaseless stomach related problems or cracked gut, the all-inclusive time of fasting may be beneficial. Considering stomach related issues are a characteristic wellspring of constant aggravation and immune system issue today, the advantages of fasting are extensive extending.

Common Intermittent Fasting Myths

In spite of the proof displaying its numerous advantages, there are as yet a few intermittent fasting myths that keep on flowing today. I am going to separate this one by one and clarify what science and the episodic proof are letting us know.

Unnatural and Unhealthy for the Body

A standout amongst the most noticeable intermittent fasting myths is the possibility that abandoning sustenance is unnatural and conceivably unsafe for the body. This may be because our built up dietary establishments have lectured three square dinners daily for such a long time. The customary conviction was that we always have to take in nourishment to keep our digestion consuming hot.

What we cannot deny is that this eating example will really will, in general, advance weight gain, sugar cravings, and mindset irregular characteristics.

Times of fasting were generally ordinary for our predecessors. We have metabolic adjustment forms that jump out at assistance we flourish through these seasons of shortage. For instance, the capacity to deliver vitality from fats means that our bodies are stable and steady to go vast stretches with no nourishment.

Intermittent fasting appears to have an overall recuperating impact on the body by animating fix and security instruments.

Hinders Your Metabolism

As was referenced effectively, a large portion of us was raised on the possibility that we need 3 square suppers daily to keep our digestion consuming and glucose stable. When these dinners are dependent on carbs and sugar as the essential wellspring of calories, in any case, this eating example will in general advance weight gain, insulin obstruction, and an increased danger of coronary illness.

Research demonstrates that intermittent fasting can have a digestion-boosting impact as it advances a condition of ketosis and increases development hormone levels. What does hinder the digestion is drawn out calorie confinement. This is the reason abstaining from excessive food intake in common sense may not be an extraordinary thought.

This is one of the discontinuous fasting legends that hold some weight yet is effectively settled. You should guarantee you are expending enough calories to fulfill the metabolic needs of your body. There are a few online apparatuses that can enable you to evaluate your metabolic rate.

Causes Nutrient Deficiencies

Fasting doesn't cause supplement lacks, supplement insufficient weight control plans do! When you are expending an excellent entire sustenances diet inside your eating window, it is far-fetched that you will experience the ill effects of any supplement insufficiencies.

If you are likewise following a ketogenic diet and additionally devouring caffeine all the time, you may need to hydrate more and expend more minerals by utilizing an astounding salt on your nourishment. I usually suggest either Himalayan pink or Celtic dim ocean salt for this.

Other than that, there is next to no explanation behind the better our insulin affectability, the less insulin our body a standout amongst the most unwarranted. When you quick, your body builds up a more noteworthy dimension of supplement proficiency. At the point when our glucose levels are going here and there, we channel quite a bit of our supplement stores. When we quick, we go through fundamentally fewer supplements and can hold them for some time later.

Causes Muscle Loss

One of the intermittent fasting myths starting from the wellness business is that intermittent fasting will prompt lost bulk. While the facts confirm that the body will inevitably return to making vitality from muscle proteins amid times of delayed caloric confinement, this is probably not going to occur amid a daily intermittent quick.

An ongoing report demonstrated that other day fasting for a time of about two months animated fat misfortune overall of 12 lbs while there was no massive misfortune in muscle mass. There is a protein saving impact of fasting routinely, possibly from the incitement of development hormone.

If calories and protein admission are advanced inside the eating window, you may have the option to lose fat and addition muscle in the meantime!

Causes Eating Disorders

Dietary issues are common in our general public. When you incline that you battle to join sound nutritional decisions on a daily premise, at that point, intermittent fasting may not be for you presently. I would prescribe starting with a mitigating nourishment plan as laid out here:

- It isn't likely that intermittent fasting would cause a dietary issue. It is conceivable that a dietary procedure went for advancing weight reduction would pull in the individuals who as of now battle with nutritional problems, nonetheless.

- To offer another viewpoint, steady fixation on nourishment and incautious dietary patterns are regularly to a great extent brought about by irregular glucose characteristics. Following a ketogenic diet while utilizing intermittent fasting can go far in busting sugar cravings.

- A few people will have the desire to overeat after their fasting window, which could likewise be viewed as a dietary issue. If your objective is weight reduction and inferring the numerous medical advantages from intermittent fasting, voraciously consuming food will hinder these advantages.

Not Good for People with Diabetes

The possibility that we have to eat continually to keep up level glucose is an intermittent fasting legend that overruns the diabetic network also. An ongoing report demonstrated that intermittent fasting improved weight reduction, fasting glucose, and settled glucose after supper in a gathering of sort two diabetics.

Delayed fasting may even have the option to reestablish insulin sensitivity in those experiencing type 2 diabetes. As an option or blend, following a ketogenic diet for a timeframe can restore insulin sensitivity also.

The better our insulin affectability, the less insulin our body should create, and the less irritation our collection will include involvement. This is significant for people with diabetes as it lessens there a danger of coronary illness and kidney disappointment.

For sort I people with diabetes who can't create their very own insulin, it is indispensable to intently screen glucose to do this right. These people may even now have the option to quick for 12 and as long as 16 hours daily depending upon how stable they can get their glucose levels.

Supports Overeating

Glucose and leptin, to a great extent, manage our eating practices. When you have glucose unsteadiness, you will ache for sustenance when it comes slamming down. If you have progressed toward becoming desensitized to leptin, you will experience considerable difficulties deciding when you have had enough to eat.

Leptin is a flagging hormone in the body that, to a great extent, controls your craving levels. Inadequate rest, stress, voraciously consuming food, and eternal calorie limitation would all be able to add to leptin opposition which will look at last add to the propensity to indulge.

Intermittent fasting improves glucose soundness and leptin sensitivity, which ought to enhance motivation command over overeating. If you are as yet attempting to beat your cravings.

The Secret to Intermittent Fasting for Women

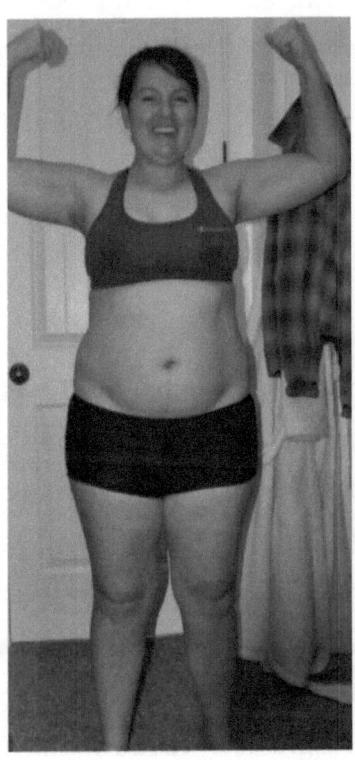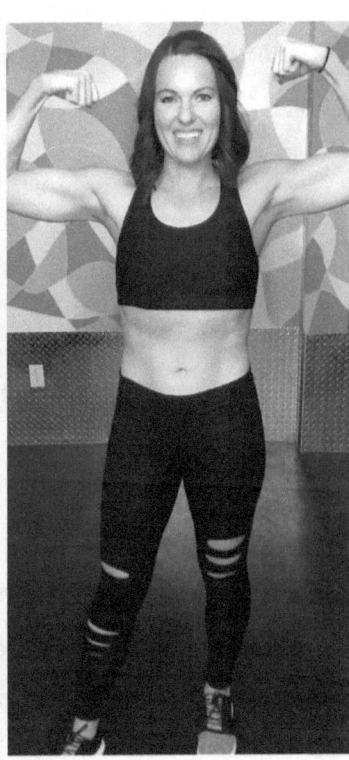

Odds are if you are wellbeing and fitness savvy, you've known about intermittent fasting and its advantages for fat misfortune and by and significant wellbeing.

However, did you realize that, in case you're a lady, fasting could prompt hormonal unevenness and could prompt fruitfulness issues if not done appropriately? Here, we'll talk about the ideal ways for ladies to appreciate the positive parts of intermittent fasting without putting their wellbeing in danger.

Why Fasting?

An intermittent fast is a concise fast where, for 12– 16 hours or more, you don't eat anything except water (a couple of exceptional cases apply). And keeping in mind that that may sound incredibly difficult to accomplish, you may as of now be fasting without knowing it in the event that you have supper at, state, 7 p.m. also, break your fast toward the beginning of the day between 7—10 a.m. — and if you just have water and dark espresso or tea between.

For others of us who have been prepared to eat six times each day to "keep our digestion up," it tends to be a challenging and conflicting accomplishment to go 12 or more hours on water alone. Science backs this antiquated practice.

Therapeutic studies have appeared intermittent fasting:

- Expands vitality

- Improves cognizance, memory and consistent discernment

- Makes us less insulin safe, fighting off fat and an insulin-related malady by diminishing dimensions of flowing IGF-1 and expanding insulin affectability without bringing down the resting metabolic rate

- May improve invulnerability, lower diabetes hazard, and strengthen heart wellbeing.

- Expands generation of cerebrum neurotropic development factor — a protein that advances neuron development and insurance — making us stronger to neurological pressure and in this manner fighting off neurodegenerative maladies.

The Fasting and Hormone Connection

Necessarily, intermittent fasting can cause hormonal irregularity in ladies if it's not done effectively. Ladies are very delicate to sign of starvation, and if the body detects that it is being famished, it will increase the generation of the yearning hormones leptin and ghrelin.

So when ladies experience voracious appetite after under-eating, they are encountering the expanded generation of these hormones. It's the female body's method for securing a potential embryo — notwithstanding when a lady isn't pregnant.

However, numerous ladies overlook these craving prompts, making the sign get significantly more intense. Or then again, increasingly awful, we attempt to disregard them, at that point fall flat and gorge later, at that point line that up with under-eating and starvation once more. Furthermore, prepare to have your mind blown. That endless loop can toss your hormones askew and even stop ovulation.

In animal studies, following two weeks of intermittent fasting, female rats quit having menstrual cycles and their ovaries contracted while encountering more a sleeping disorder than their male partners (however the male rats experienced lower testosterone generation). Tragically, there are not very many human studies taking a gander at the contrasts between intermittent fasting for people, however the animal studies affirm our doubt: Intermittent fasting for significant lots of time can at times lose a lady's hormonal equalization, cause ripeness issues and worsen dietary problems like anorexia, bulimia and voraciously consuming food issue.

Crescendo Fasting for Women

Intermittent fasting for ladies can be challenging for your body if you are unfamiliar to it or when you bounce in too rapidly. So if you are a lady or having a go at fasting out of the blue, you may profit by adjusted — or crescendo — intermittent fasting.

Crescendo fasting expects you to fast a couple of days seven days rather than consistently. My experience is that ladies get significantly more profit by doing it along these lines without incidentally tossing their hormones into free for all. This is a progressively delicate methodology that helps the body all the more effectively adjust to fasting. What's more, if ladies do it right, it very well may be an astounding method to shave off muscle versus fat, improve fiery markers and addition vitality.

Not all ladies need crescendo fasting, yet it will guarantee accomplishment in most.

Standards of Crescendo Fasting:

- Fast on 2– 3 nonconsecutive days out of every week (for example Tuesday, Thursday and Saturday)

- On fasting days, do yoga or light cardio.

- Ideally, fast for 12– 16 hours.

- Eat regularly on your quality preparing/HIIT exercises exceptional exercise days.

- Drink a lot of water. (Tea and espresso are alright, as well, insofar as there is no added milk or sugar)

- Following two weeks, don't hesitate to include one more day of fasting.

Discretionary: Consider taking 5– 8 grams of BCAAs amid your fast. A stretched chain amino corrosive enhancement has a couple of calories yet gives fuel to muscles. This can offer some relief from appetite and weariness.

When you have fizzled at intermittent fasting previously, attempt this crescendo style for a superior, progressively practical experience — mainly if you are a lady.

CHAPTER TWO

The Pros and Cons of Intermittent Fasting

Registered dietitians take on one of the most talked about weight loss trends.

For a great many people, the word fasting raises the thought of delayed periods without sustenance or possibly drink. A few people fast intermittently for religious reasons or therapeutic need (say, before a methodology). Another eating regimen has individuals fasting to get in shape, improve health, live more (and healthier), help mental clarity, and the sky is the limit from there. This is the thing that you need to consider this trendy fast.

Intermittent fasting might be rehearsed in a couple of various ways, as indicated by research regarding the matter:

Substitute day fasting is exactly what it sounds like. On exchanging days, you either gala or fast.

Altered fasting, otherwise called 5:2 intermittent fasting, includes eating typically five days seven days with nourishment confined to about 25% of your calorie needs on two non-successive days. (Think: around 500 calories or less on confined days.)

Time confined fasting limits nourishment inside exact time windows, express 8 PM to 10 AM. In this kind of fasting, you go 12 to 16 hours restricting nourishment.

Will you get thinner?

These types of fasting do seem to advance weight misfortune. In any case, the science is slight among people, and average examinations include little example sizes and constrained spans. In any case, the results recommend that individuals do get in shape, so, if you need to give it a go, this is what you should know.

How does intermittent fasting work?

There are a couple of things impacting everything. Your circadian check is effectively engaged with managing your digestion and various hormones, including the craving controlling hormones leptin and ghrelin, are liable to these day/night designs. Studies have demonstrated that eating most of the nourishment prior in the day adjusts all the more intimately with our circadian rhythms, and disturbing these rhythms by eating late around evening time or state, eating as per move work, prompts a higher post-feast glucose reaction, delayed insulin introduction, and a more severe danger of sort 2 diabetes and stoutness.

Past this current, there's a social segment at play. Late night nibbling can be a common practice (as any of us who have cozied up to a bowl of popcorn knows), and setting up standards to balance this helps limit gorging.

At last, poor rest quality and getting deficient rest is a realized hazard factor for weight, and by limiting evening eating (and in this manner, lessening acid reflux), you could get more rest and the rest you get may even be increasingly acceptable, which certainly brings health benefits.

What is a portion of the drawbacks of intermittent fasting?

A few examinations locate a higher drop out appropriate among intermittent fasters, which recommends it probably won't be a feasible methodology. Besides, it may have different results. If, for example, you're doing exchange day fasting and everything you can consider on your fasting days is sustenance that can meddle with a center, and possibly your hands on execution. Additionally, there might be social ramifications to intermittent fasting. Are your companions gathering for supper at 7 and you're cut off from nourishment at 6? You can perceive how this could meddle with your public activity.

There might be medicinal worries too. In this year-long investigation, unhealthy LDL cholesterol had expanded fundamentally following a year among the other fasting gathering. This may spell inconvenience for your heart.

At last, I've known about individuals utilizing their non-fasting days to top off on sustenances, similar to pizza, fatty sweets, French fries and another charge that is low in nourishment and doesn't fuel a healthy body. Although you may at present get more fit because of the calorie deficiencies on different days, you won't get the defensive advantages of sound sustenance.

Who can profit by intermittent fasting?

In case you're a devotee of a win big or bust methodology, or in case you're somebody who likes characterized principles to pursue, intermittent fasting could merit attempting. It likewise may be particularly useful for individuals who take an interest in mindless eating during the evening since the hard stop will check this conduct.

Who shouldn't attempt intermittent fasting?

Try not to endeavor to fast when you've had a dietary issue or indications of scattered eating, which incorporate (yet aren't constrained to) voraciously consuming food, sustenance fixation, abuse of laxatives and outrageous nourishment confinement. In case you're pregnant or bosom encouraging, you ought not to endeavor intermittent fasting. Anybody being treated for diabetes (with prescriptions) just as anybody with disease and those with a bargained insusceptible framework ought to likewise maintain a strategic distance from intermittent fasting (or address their specialist before attempting it).

What should you know before you give it go?

If you do attempt it, make the most of your calories by picking healthy sustenances that work admirably topping you off. Concentrate on an assortment of veggies to ensure you get a variety of healthy mixes, alongside quality protein sources, (for example, eggs, skinless poultry, fish and other fish), which work superbly keeping yearning under control. Offset out your suppers with foods grown from the ground grains. In case you're completing another fasting diet, you'll need to give close consideration to bring down calorie sustenances that make volume — both on your plate and in your gut. Keep in mind, similarly as with any reasonable eating plan, non-boring vegetables are your companions.

What's more, remember, it is anything but an enchantment slug. Specialists trust that the genuine key to enduring weight lies by the way you handle the upkeep stage. "It is difficult, however many individuals do effectively get in shape," "You have to focus on what you eat, the amount you eat, and how you're supporting that procedure — either with a gathering or a companion or a healthcare expert to keep you responsible and help you deal with the ordinary slip-ups that are a piece of life."

Intermittent Fasting Pros and Cons

With the expansion in the measure of proof of the conflicting results of being overweight, a developing extent of society is winding up more wellbeing cognizant. To deal with their weight, many are adopting diets and different preparing techniques, for example, intermittent fasting.

Moving far from conventional calorie restriction, intermittent fasting has turned out to be progressively mainstream as of late. What are the advantages and outcomes of following such an arrangement?

What is Intermittent Fasting?

There are a few kinds of intermittent fasting which might be separated by the dimension of calorie restriction and the recurrence of eating. For a few, intermittent fasting is a piece of their religion; for instance, Muslims can't devour any nourishment or drink among daybreak and nightfall amid the long stretch of Ramadan. The absolute most basic kinds of intermittent fasting are laid out beneath.

Kinds of Intermittent Fasting

Interchange Day Fasting (ADF)

ADF is intermittent fasting that requires one "feed day" where those following the eating regimen can eat at whatever point and anything they desire inside 24 hours. This is rotated with a "quick day" where you're unfit to consume for a limit of 24 hours. There are varieties of ADF which may make it simpler to pursue, for example, enabling a limit of 500 calories to be devoured on "quick days." On quick days, those following the eating routine can drink no-calorie refreshments, for example, tea, espresso, and water. Notwithstanding, the utilization of sugars, sugar, or cream with hot beverages isn't prescribed.

Adjusted Fasting Regimens

On adjusted fasting regimens, the individuals who tail them are permitted to eat sustenance normally, yet are confined to devouring just around 20-25% of the required energy on fasting days. This program shapes the premise of the prominent 5:2 eating regimen, which recommends energy restriction on two days of the week while on the staying five days, the typical calorie admission is permitted.

Time-Restricted Feeding

Those following the time-confined sustaining routine are permitted to eat whatever they like, however rather than calorie restriction, they are limited to eating inside determined timeframes. The period can go from 6 to 12 hours, and outside of this window, just the utilization of no-calorie beverages and water is allowed.

Experts of Intermittent Fasting

A few sorts of intermittent fasting have been related to various advantages for their disciples contrasted with other customary diets.

Weight reduction

One of the primary reasons why individuals receive intermittent fasting is to oversee or shed pounds. Proof proposes that intermittent fasting can be beneficial as a weight reduction device. Explicit research exploring the impacts of ADF on weight reduction found that inside a 2 to the three weeks, there was a 2.5% decrease in weight contrasted with gauge estimations.

Medical advantages

It has been discovered that intermittent fasting can have a few long haul protection medical advantages. It is all around looked into that being overweight and hefty can improve the probability of building up a scope of serious sicknesses; for example, coronary supply route malady (CAD). An intermittent fasting dietary program would thus be able to achieve a decrease in triacylglycerol focuses, and expansion in high-thickness lipoprotein cholesterol. These progressions lead to a general reduction in the danger of creating CAD. Further research has additionally shown that by adopting intermittent fasting, individuals can decrease the probability of creating age-related maladies, for example, Alzheimer's.

It's simpler to pursue

Research has discovered that individuals think that it's more straightforward to pursue an intermittent fasting diet over a long haul period contrasted with following a calorie-confined eating routine. It is recommended that as individuals need to diminish their calorie admission each other day on the ADF diet, it is simpler to accomplish than bringing down utilization consistently. Indeed, even the individuals who pursue the altered ADF diet, where they can expend 500 calories on "quick days," have discovered considerably more feasible than keeping up a steady calorie shortfall. Like this, for those needing to accomplish possible weight reduction, intermittent fasting may be extremely beneficial.

Cons of Intermittent Fasting

The individuals who are considering adopting intermittent fasting into their routine might need to think about the accompanying negatives.

Symptoms of Intermittent Fasting

In the same way as other diets, intermittent fasting can have a few reactions. Research exploring the effect of ADF on weight reduction found that participants experienced headaches, constipation, and absence of energy. The announced lack of power might be an issue for those wishing to prepare or work out, which is additionally prescribed for grown-ups to keep up a sound way of life.

Besides, changing mental impacts were accounted for, for example, an absence of fixation and awful temper. One unique feature from the exploration was that individuals were observed to be progressively distracted with sustenance because of intermittent fasting. This may bring on additional issues for the individuals who are inclined to specific dietary problems.

The Effectiveness of Intermittent Fasting in Weight Loss

There are clashing examination discoveries on the effect of intermittent fasting on weight reduction contrasted with conventional calorie confined diets. A few specialists recommend that intermittent fasting isn't better than typical calorie-limited foods.

Suitability of Intermittent Fasting

Regardless of the numerous medical advantages that it offers for individuals who are overweight, fat or of healthy weight, intermittent fasting isn't reasonable for everybody. There are explicit gatherings of society for whom this arrangement isn't prescribed, for example, pregnant ladies, those with dietary issues and those with some medical issues.

Intermittent Fasting For Weight Loss Tips

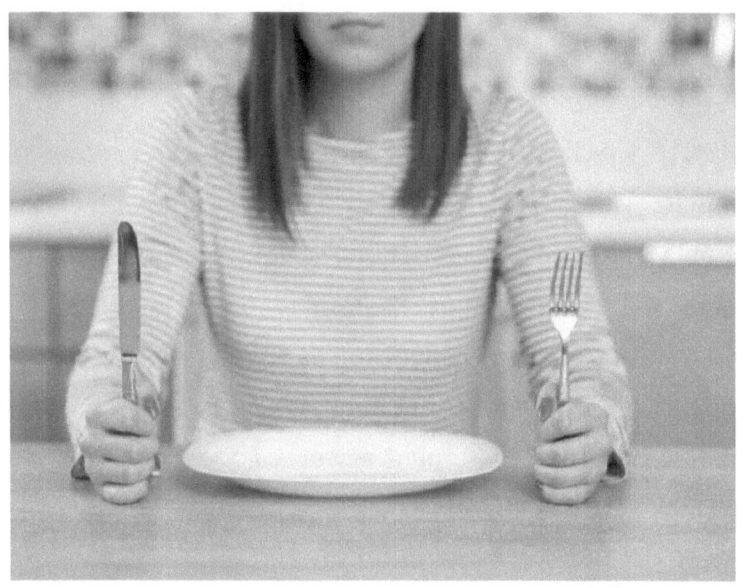

There's no uncertainty about it that an ever increasing number of people today are utilizing intermittent fasting for weight loss. In case you don't know what intermittent fasting is, It's mainly when you deliberately use times of fasting to drive your body into consuming fat as a fuel source. This method of weight loss is very compelling;

however, you need to ensure you're doing it right or else you can, in reality, moderate your digestion.

While you are experiencing a fasting period, you should devour water alongside Branched Chain Amino Acids (BCAA) which will help counteract the breakdown of muscle. This might be unreasonably extreme for certain people since you will no doubt experience hunger, and there will be an abnormal state of order important for intermittent fasting. The individuals who are for this kind of weight loss guarantee that they can get results snappier than customary consuming fewer calories practices, for example, calorie limitation.

If you're new to intermittent fasting, at that point, it's suggested that you complete time for testing of 24 hours to ensure you can proceed with doing these for an all-encompassing timeframe. It will be reasonable to become easily irritable towards people amid your fasting day, so get ready for the most exceedingly awful. I want to have a cheat day before the fasting day, so I can set up my body for the quick and furthermore quicken the outcomes. The enormous caloric admission of the cheat day primes my body to consume progressively fat as a fuel source on the fasting day.

I additionally personally want to utilize Sundays as my fasting days since I have minimal measure of connection with society because by and by it's anything but difficult to become irritable. Make sure to take your BCAA's for the day in 5-10 gram servings like you would set up for standard suppers. In the end, after you have expertly finished the 24 hours fasts, you can advance to further developed methods of intermittent fasting, for example, utilizing numerous ones consistently.

Intermittent fasting won't be for everyone except if you're not kidding about getting some excellent outcomes; at that point, this will support them. Everyone should, in any case, become familiar with the nuts and bolts of a healthy eating routine and exercise program. You can exercise on your fasting days to upgrade the fat loss, yet it will be challenging for some to gather the vitality to do as such. By and large, ensure you prepare to precede your fasting day as it will be instrumental in your prosperity with the program.

Intermittent Fasting For Weight Loss - A Simple Solution to Burn Off Fat

There are numerous approaches to get in shape, and every person has an example of overcoming the adversity of their own. When I get some information about the kinds of things they have attempted to diminish their body fat rate, I frequently get told that intermittent fasting for weight loss is a feasible thought. Without a doubt, doubtlessly the rationale behind this methodology might be spot on track - anyway how about we did not bounce to that determination before we complete a touch of an investigation.

Firstly, if we are to demonstrate that intermittent fasting for weight loss does undoubtedly work, we have to explain that the hypothesis could without a doubt prove to be useful in the objective of losing overabundance weight. If we eat, stop and after that eat again over the time of a month or something like that - what would we be able to anticipate? As I would see it, I would hope to see mellow weight loss, however positively not outcomes. We as a whole realize that to get in shape and keep it off, we have to accelerate the digestion while decreasing the measure of vitality we are expanding. This is regularly a delicate balance to accomplish - as the general thought of developing the metabolism requires extra exercise, which results in a prerequisite for more vitality admission.

This is, to some degree, a difficult predicament. It might appear to be then that intermittent fasting is the answer to this issue. If one somehow managed to substitute times of eating with times of starvation, while practicing all through the whole time frame - the digestion may get a kick all through the entire time the method was being utilized. It ought to be referenced anyway that a few people will observe various outcomes to other people. All in all, the standard of fasting appears to be a decent one. Similarly, as with any eating routine, however - counsel a medicinal expert first.

Fasting Benefits - Using Intermittent Fasting For Weight Loss Effectively

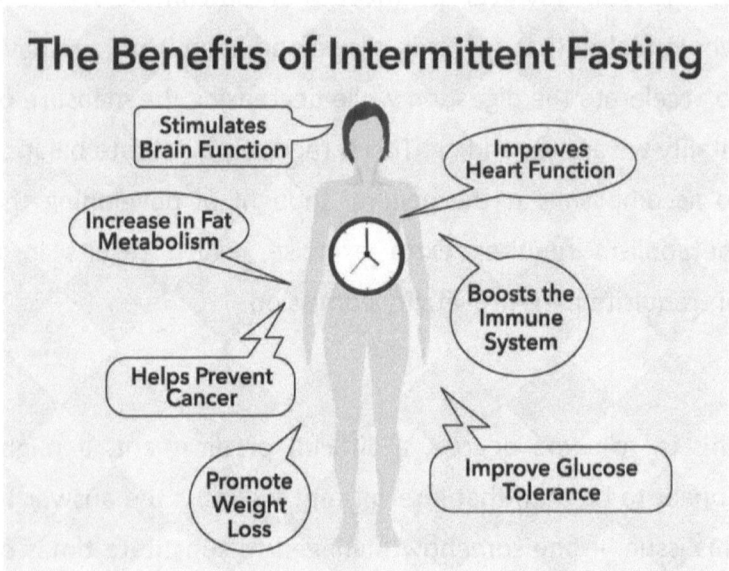

First of all, to have the option to apply for the fasting benefits, we should first comprehend the idea of fasting for weight loss.

Things being what they are, what is fasting? It is fundamentally the procedure of cognizant refusing nourishment and beverages (aside from water) for a specific timeframe.

Fasting has been around for quite a long time, utilized with various capacities, and has become fairly prominent in recent years, and above all as fasting for weight loss. The reason for that was a contextual investigation, with no exclusive standards at first, which was made on people fasting for a year or more. As I stated, they didn't expect much from It, yet the outcomes were so astounding, a more profound examination was required.

As fasting benefits, people wound up getting thinner, improving their medical issues. When they had a few, frequently. They additionally said to look more youthful and even have a more extended and more joyful life! This is the reason this method is so captivating to me. It's a similar motivation behind why I need to share the intermittent fasting benefits with you.

In reality, this eating design isn't that convoluted. Essentially what you do is eat amid 24 hours as you wish, at that point the following 24 hours you quick. This implies no sustenance! (Separated from water). It is altogether different from our regular eating habits. Although it might appear as an extreme weight loss method, fasting for weight loss is upheld by science to be the best and characteristic a long distance!

Here are the primary three intermittent fastings for weight loss benefits that emerge the most:

- Detoxification - It is a standout amongst the most significant fasting advantages of all. As you quick, experiences a self-cleaning process, when liberated from steady nourishment preparing. This enables it to clear out your body toxins accumulated amid overwhelming snacks or swift, inexpensive food dinners. Furthermore, from that point onward, you feel simply extraordinary!

- Developing tolerance - Most people will, in general neglect this tremendous fasting advantage. Lamentably, a large portion of us does not have this vital quality, amid eating regimens, however, for the most part in everyday life. Patience originates from discretion, and this one resembles a muscle: the more you train it, the more grounded it gets. In this way, alongside other fasting benefits, you likewise become more grounded rationally!

- Effective weight loss! These days it's the principle fasting advantage, and the fundamental motivation behind why the vast majority get into it is fasting for weight loss. In reality, our bodies are intended to live long without sustenance, as we did in the senior days. When we eat, our liver and muscles store vitality as glycogen. In the fasting days, our body uses glycogen first for two or three hours; at that point, it begins consuming off the fat.

These fasting benefits are only general ones. Aside from these, every person experiences his very own advantages from the way toward fasting, because every one of us is one of a kind. What's more, indeed, every last one of us has the right to be in the shape that the person needs to be! Good karma!

CHAPTER THREE

How to do Intermittent Fasting for Women Over 40

Intermittent fasting for ladies is a viable weight reduction approach, particularly ladies more than 40. As ladies age, I am getting thinner turns out to be increasingly testing. Intermittent fasting gives a simple method for ladies to get leaner and accomplish extraordinary wellbeing. This section will detail the particular advantages of intermittent fasting for ladies more than 40.

What is Intermittent Fasting?

Intermittent fasting (IF) alludes to an eating design which causes you to cycle between times of eating and fasting. It doesn't say much regarding the sort of sustenances to incorporate into your eating routine arrangement yet centers around when you ought to eat them.

There are various approaches to perform intermittent fasting, all of which split the days into eating and fasting periods. In spite of what individuals regularly accept, intermittent fasting is, in reality, simple to do.

Advantages of Intermittent Fasting for Women Over 40

The benefits of intermittent fasting for ladies are settled and Science-sponsored. For what reason is it explicitly valuable for ladies more than 40?

Weight reduction

Weight reduction is among the top advantages of intermittent fasting for ladies more than 40. There are declarations wherever about how intermittent fasting has helped individuals lose considerable measures of weight. There are likewise scholastic examinations that help this idea.

Bringing down Cancer Risk

When has demonstrated to be a significant prognostic device against malignancy, the underlying proof has discovered that the demonstration of fasting represses specific pathways that may change some way or another lead to the advancement and movement of malignant growth.

Decreasing Diabetes Risk

The danger of diabetes, which uniquely elevates amid middle age, can be effectively controlled through intermittent fasting. It does as such by bringing down insulin level and controlling insulin obstruction in the body.

Hostile to maturing

It has been accounted for to hinder the improvement of diseases that lead to death, intermittent fasting for ladies more than 40 can provide assistance they carry on with a more drawn out, more advantageous life when contrasted with the individuals who pursue a customary eating regimen plan.

Heart Health

It is typical for your cardiovascular wellbeing to begin declining around age 40. If can help hinder this weakening and avoid certain cardiovascular diseases like hypertension by bringing down LDL cholesterol and triglycerides.

Diminished Inflammation

Ceaseless aggravation harms your body, making it harder to shed pounds. Following intermittent fasting, turns around nuisance and may improve your general prosperity.

Muscle Preservation

One of the advantages of following IF is that it encourages you to lose more weight while holding bulk. A higher quantity, like this, causes you to consume more calories, notwithstanding when you are not engaged with physical exercises.

Diminished Cravings

Another advantage of intermittent fasting for ladies more than 40 is diminished longings. Changing to this eating regimen adjusts your dietary patterns and typically help you eat lesser than expected. These reductions the quantity of calories expended every day and subsequently, diminishes body weight.

Improvement in Mental Health

In the off chance that in females have been gotten a kick out of the opportunity of neurogenesis: the procedure wherein new cerebrum cells are created. Neurogenesis, at last, expands your cerebrum performance, center, disposition, and memory.

Sorts of Intermittent Fasting

Since you think about the benefits of intermittent fasting for ladies more than 40, you should need to think about the various kinds of IF.

16/8 Daily Fasting

The 16/8 technique incorporates fasting each day for 14 to 16 hours with an eating window of 8 to 10 hours. Inside this eating window, you can without much of a stretch fit 2 to 3 suppers.

For instance, if you eat your last supper at 8 pm and don't eat whatever else until noon the following morning, you are fasting for 16 hours in a row. Amid the fasting hours, you are permitted to drink espresso, water, and non-caloric refreshments.

Ladies are by and large prescribed too quick for 14 to 15 hours.

5:2 Fasting

The 5:2 eating regimen incorporates eating ordinarily for five days seven days while confining your caloric admission to 500-600 for the staying two days. On the fasting days, it is prescribed for ladies to eat 500 calories.

For example, you can eat typically on all days except Mondays and Thursdays. On these two days, you can eat two little dinners, each will 250 calories.

Eat Stop Eat

The Eat-Stop-Eat approach expects you to watch a 24-hour long quick on more than one occasion per week. You can begin fasting from supper on the very first moment and prop it up till supper time the next day.

For example, if you take your keep going supper on Monday at 7 pm and don't eat anything until 7 pm Tuesday, you have quite recently watched an entire 24-hour quick. Additionally, you can use likewise quick from breakfast to breakfast, or from lunch to lunch. The final product would not adjust.

You can drink non-caloric refreshments, for example, water and espresso amid the fasting hours. No substantial sustenance is permitted.

Intermittent Fasting for Women: Balancing Hormones and Crescendo Fasting

change and could cause issues if not went into appropriately. This is particularly valid if you hop in too forcefully toward the start; additionally, I can now and then reason hormonal irregularity in females if it isn't watched appropriately.

This is because ladies will, in general, be incredibly touchy to the sign of starvation. If their body detects that it is in a condition of hunger, it will expand the creation of craving hormone ghrelin and leptin, prompting food cravings.

You may disregard these food cravings, yet this will result in an endless loop that will rattle your hormones.

Thus, if you are a female more than 40 who are attempting IF out of the blue, it is smarter, to begin with, Crescendo Fasting.

Crescendo fasting expects you to quick for a couple of days out of each week rather than every day. It is especially useful for ladies to get in shape without aggravating hormones. Whenever done right, Crescendo IF can be an incredible method to shed body weight, gain vitality, and improve incendiary markers.

To pursue Crescendo fasting, you have to quick on 2-3 non-sequential days of the week, for instance, Monday, Wednesday, and Friday. It is prescribed to perform aerobic exercises or light cardio on the fasting days.

On your quality preparing or progressively thorough exercise days, you should eat regularly. Make sure that you drink a lot of water and some other refreshment with no added milk or sugar. After following the Crescendo fasting for about fourteen days, you can add another fasting day to your week after week plan.

Exceptional Tips for Intermittent Fasting and Women Over 40

The benefits of intermittent fasting for ladies more than 40 are various. Ensure you get the vast majority of these advantages by following these extra tips.

Favor Salads

Raw vegetables are an extraordinary wellspring of nutrients, phytonutrients, minerals, and other helpful substances. Also, they are additionally ordinarily high in cell reinforcements that ensure your body against free extreme harm.

In this way, take a stab at breaking your quick with a significant bowl of salad containing crisp green vegetables like kale, romaine lettuce, or Swiss chard. Toss in sure cucumbers, tomatoes, and a few avocados to get solid fats. Utilize olive oil as a dressing, and voila, you have a delicious homemade salad right before you.

Amid eating, window eats sustenances high in fiber.

Fiber is an extraordinary substance for stomach related wellbeing. When you eat nourishments high in fiber, for instance, entire grains and beans, the sugar in these sustenances are economically retained into the blood. This guarantees your blood glucose levels don't rise excessively quick.

For what reason is this useful? Since sudden spikes in blood glucose will in general fall quickly, making you feel hungry not long after you have eaten. This inevitably leads to indulging.

Likewise, fiber additionally upgrades your metabolic rate to advance weight reduction. So remember to incorporate fiber-rich nourishments in your eating window.

Begin with Crescendo Fasting

As referenced previously, ladies are increasingly touchy to fasting since fasting directly affects their body hormones. This can adjust their body capacities and lead to various menstrual issues.

Since Crescendo fasting is uncommonly planned to enable ladies to watch IF without causing irregular hormonal characteristics, ensure you embrace this technique for fasting as you start your IF venture.

Screen your Hormones Closely

While following IF, make sure to give a nearby consideration to how your hormones are reacting to the adjustments in eating regimen. A portion of the hormones that you should watch out for include:

- Insulin
- Ghrelin
- Leptin
- Estrogen
- Progesterone
- Realize When to Stop

When you begin feeling any unusual symptoms, quit fasting quickly, and contact your doctor. A portion of the signs to pay unique mind to include:

- Expanded feelings of anxiety
- Male pattern baldness

- Low vitality
- Emotional episodes
- Sadness or tension
- Muscle torment
- Loss of menstrual cycle
- Loss of charisma
- Extra Weight Loss Tips for Women Over 40

To ensure you lose the most critical measure of weight most productively, pursue these extra tips.

Get Enough Sleep

Short rest has been connected to expanded appetite and weight gain since it exasperates leptin and ghrelin-the two important hormones controlling yearning. So hold these hormones under tight restraints by ensuring you rest 8 hours per day.

Quality Train

As you age, your body will, in general, lose muscle. The best way to get it back is to quality train. So gear up and agree to accept a weight instructional meeting. The sooner you start, the better.

Eat Less Sugar

As you age, you will, in general, become progressively impervious to insulin; for example, you experience difficulty retaining glucose. Expending sugary sustenances in such circumstances leads to the aggregation of glucose in the body, causing a ton of dangers. So eliminated everything that has sugar in it.

Keep a Food Journal

Keep a sustenance diary to record your week after week dietary patterns. This will enable you to monitor what you are eating and may allow you to choose which nourishments are hurting you.

Take a Probiotic

Probiotics are robust microbes found in your gut. Taking these enhancements will improve your absorption and progress in general wellbeing.

21 Day Intermittent Fasting PLAN

Step by step instructions to begin discontinuous fasting

To successfully begin with Intermittent Fasting, it is essential to comprehend the different sorts of Intermittent Fasting. That is the way you will locate the one that works the best for you and accommodates your excellent way of life.

Here are the most mainstream Intermittent Fasting Schedules.

- Irregular fasting 16/8

- How: Fast for 16 h and Eat eighth

By following this 16/8 Intermittent Fasting Schedule, you quick for 16 hours and confine your eating to an 8-hour eating window.

You can adjust the calendar as per your way of life, notwithstanding, most practitioners quick from supper to noon – which implies just skipping breakfast. Significant is to keep up a reliable eating time.

Irregular FASTING 5:2 a.k.a The Fast Diet

How: 2 days of the week limit calories to 500-600, five days out of each week eat typically

5:2 Intermittent Fasting gives you a chance to eat regularly five days out of each week and limits your calorie admission to 500-600 every day amid the other two days. While picking your fasting days, remember that there ought to be in any event one regular eating day in the middle.

If you will probably get in shape, it is critical to stick to smart dieting on the five days amid which you are not fasting.

- Discontinuous fasting 20/4 A.K.A. WARRIOR DIET

- How: Fast for 20 h and Eat for 4h.

As opposed to different strategies, while following 20/4 Intermittent Fasting Schedule, you are permitted to eat some crude products of the soil, and some lean protein amid the 20 hr quick time frame.

The 4-hour eating window will be at night and you ought to pursue an unusual request of eating exact nutrition types: beginning with vegetables, proteins and fat, and eating carbs just if you are as yet ravenous.

- Practicing will be done in a fasted state.

- 24 HR FAST A.K.A. EAT STOP EAT

- How: Fast for 24 h 1-2 times each week

While following 24 hours quick, you should quick for 24 hours 1-2 days a week and eat regularly on different days. That way, you ought to diminish by, and large calorie consumption by 10%, and consequently get in shape.

Prescribed Intermittent Fasting Schedule

Other than the recently mentioned, there are different Intermittent Fasting types like One Meal a Day (OMAD) and numerous sorts of delayed fasting.

For our test, we prescribe the most well-known strategy – Intermittent Fasting 16/8.

16/8 additionally happens to be the most prominent strategy among famous people. When you are interested to know how they work on fasting and what are the principle benefits (Coldplay soloist Chris Martin trusts Intermittent Fasting encourages him to sing better!), look at our blog entry on How to do Intermittent Fasting According to 40 Famous People.

what to eat amid discontinuous fasting?

A well-known misguided judgment is that you can enable yourself to eat anything while at the same time doing Intermittent Fasting, including cheap food, sugary, and exceptionally prepared dishes. When you will likely shed pounds, improve productivity, and get more advantageous, it is critical to stick to sound dinners.

This implies entire eating sustenances and maintaining a strategic distance from the standard speculates, for example, sugar, handled nourishments, void carbs, and so forth.

The eating regimen you pick is up to you, as long it is adjusted and accommodates your way of life. For some, Keto Diet has demonstrated to be a great supplement to Intermittent Fasting as it might enable you to consume progressively fat.

Still not sure how to execute another more beneficial eating regimen to help your Intermittent Fasting objectives and make your Intermittent Fasting venture simpler?

what to drink amid discontinuous fasting?

To get all the medical advantages of Intermittent Fasting, for example, fat misfortune, expanded metabolic rate, lower glucose levels, help in the robust framework and others, you need to limit from devouring any caloric nourishment. However, you can, at present, consume non-caloric beverages since they don't break you're quick and enable you to get every one of the advantages of fasting.

This is because non-caloric beverages don't cause the arrival of insulin, and as a result, don't meddle with fat consuming as well as autophagy (cell cleanup).

This would include:

- Water
- Shining water
- Mineral water
- Plain dark espresso
- Plain tea

Benefits of Intermittent Fasting for Women Over 50

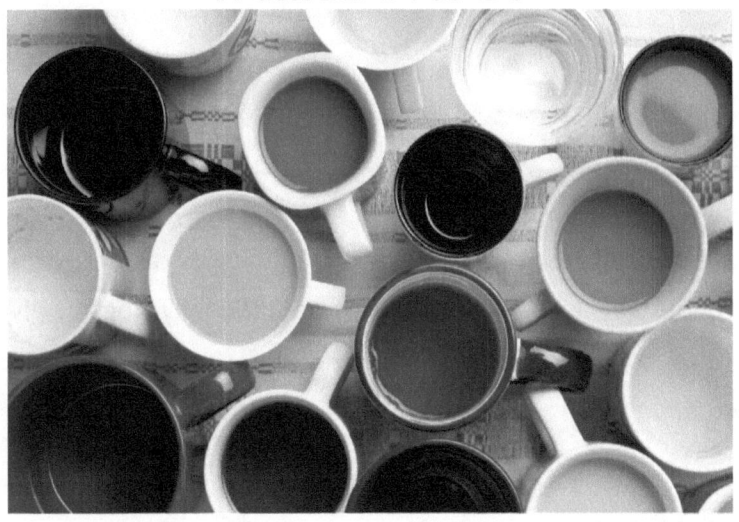

A couple of things that make it harder to get in shape after age 50 incorporate lower digestion, throbbing joints, decreased bulk, and even rest issues. In the meantime, losing fat, particularly dangerous belly fat, can significantly lessen your hazard for such genuine medical problems as diabetes, heart assaults, and malignancy.

As you age, the hazard for creating numerous maladies increments. At times, intermittent fasting for ladies more than 50 could fill in as a virtual wellspring of youth with regards to weight loss and limiting the opportunity of growing commonly age-related ailments.

How Does Intermittent Fasting Work?

Intermittent fasting, frequently alluded to as though, won't compel you to starve yourself. It additionally doesn't give you a permit to expend loads of unfortunate food amid when you don't get quick. Rather than eating suppers and snacks throughout the day, you eat inside a particular window of time.

A great many people make an IF plan that expects them to be quick for 12 to 16 hours per day. Amid the remainder of the time, they eat typical suppers and tidbits. Adhering to this eating window isn't as hard at it sounds because a great many people rest for around eight of their fasting hours. What's more, you're urged to appreciate zero-calorie drinks, similar to water, tea, and espresso.

You ought to build up an eating plan that works for you for the best discontinuous fasting results. For instance:

Twelve-hour fasts: With a 12-12 quick, you may skip breakfast and hang tight to have until lunch. If you want to eat your morning feast, you could eat an early dinner and abstain from night snacks. More seasoned ladies discover a 12-12 quick truly simple to stick to.

Sixteen-hour fasts: You may appreciate quicker outcomes with a 16-8 IF timetable. A great many people devour two dinners and a tidbit or two every day inside an eight-hour window. For instance, you may set your eating window among early afternoon and eight at night or between eight toward the beginning of the day and four toward the evening.

Five-two timetable: Restricted eating periods may not work for you consistently. Another option is to adhere to a twelve-or sixteen-hour quick for five days and after that loosen up your calendar for two days. For instance, you may utilize IF amid the week and eat regularly at the end of the week.

Every other day fasts: Another variety calls for limited calories on substitute days. For instance, you may hold your calories under 500 on one day and after that eat regularly the following day. Note that day by day IF fasts never call for limiting calories that low.

Likewise, with any eating regimen, you'll get the best outcomes in case you're predictable. In the meantime, you can unquestionably offer yourself a reprieve from this eating plan on unique events. You should test to make sense of which some kind of intermittent fasting works the best for you. Heaps of individuals slide themselves into IF with the 12-12 plan, and after that they advancement to 16-8. From that point forward, you should endeavor to adhere to that arrangement; however, much as could reasonably be expected.

What Makes Intermittent Fasting Work?

A few people trust that IF has worked for them just because the limited eating window naturally encourages them to decrease the measure of calories they expend. For instance, rather than eating three suppers and two tidbits, they may find that they possess energy for two dinners and one bite. They become progressively careful about the sorts of food they expand and will, in general, stay path from handled carbs, unwanted fat, and void calories.

You can likewise pick the sorts of healthy food that you appreciate. While a few people elect to decrease their general calorie consumption, others consolidate IF with a keto, vegetarian, or different sorts of weight control plans.

Advantages of Intermittent Fasting for Women May Extend Beyond Calorie Restriction

While some sustenance specialists battle that IF works since it helps individuals naturally limit food consumption, others oppose this idea. They trust that irregular fasting results are better than run of the mill feast plans with a similar measure of calories and different supplements. Studies have even suggested that going without food for a few hours daily accomplishes something beyond limit the measure of calories you expend.

These are some metabolic changes that IF causes that may help represent synergistic advantages:

- **Insulin:** During the fasting time frame, lower insulin levels will help improve fat consuming.

- **HGH:** While insulin levels drop, HGH levels ascend to energize fat consuming and muscle development.

- **Noradrenaline:** in light of an empty belly, the sensory system will send this concoction to cells to tell them they have to discharge fat for fuel.

Is Intermittent Fasting Healthy?

Is intermittent fasting safe? Keep in mind that you're just expected to quick for twelve to sixteen hours and not for a considerable length of time at once. Regardless you have a lot of time to appreciate a great and reliable eating routine. Some more seasoned ladies may need to eat often in light of metabolic issue or the directions on remedies. You ought to talk about your dietary patterns with your medicinal supplier before rolling out any improvements.

While it's not in fact fasting, a few specialists have detailed discontinuous fasting benefits by permitting such simple to-process food as entire natural product amid the fasting window. Modifications like these can, in any case, give your stomach related and metabolic framework a required rest. For instance, "Fit forever" was a favorite weight loss book that suggested eating just organic product after dinner and before lunch.

Run of the mill Intermittent Fasting Results

It's challenging to discover any drawbacks to IF in therapeutic writing. She clarified that amid the fasting time frame, your glucose and insulin levels would drop too low dimensions. Without insulin's hormonal fat-putting away sign, your body will depend upon put away fat for vitality.

You can likewise discover a diagram of ladies' wellbeing related irregular quick outcomes distributed by the National Library of Medicine. A few features of this report incorporate studies on the utilization of fasting as a device to decrease the danger of malignant growth, diabetes and other metabolic infections, and coronary illness.

Is Intermittent Fasting the Best Fat-Loss Tool for You?

Regardless, IF seems to work for the most part since individuals discover it genuinely simple to hold fast to, they state it encourages them to naturally limit calories and settle on better food choices by diminishing eating windows. A few studies suggest that IF is better than just cutting calories, carbs, or fat since it seems to advance fat loss while saving fit bulk.

The vast majority use IF with another weight-loss plan. For instance, you may choose to eat 1,200 calories every day to get in shape. You may think that it's a lot simpler to spread out 1,200 calories inside two suppers and two snacks than in three dinners and three tidbits. If you've battled with weight loss because you're eating regimen either didn't work or was inherently too tricky to even think about sticking to, you may attempt intermittent fasting for snappier outcomes.

CHAPTER FOUR

7 Practical Reminders for Every Woman Going Through Menopause

Menopause implies a variety of things to ladies. For a few, it's the finish of a period of childrearing and ripeness. For other people, it's a marker of the progression of time. Furthermore, for a couple of, it might even be a consequence of medical procedure or difficulties that introduce "the change."

Regardless of what menopause intends to you, odds are you will manage a portion of the side effects it brings. Here are a couple of proposals for discovering help, because occasionally even the littlest things can have the most significant impact.

1. Keep yourself cool

Night sweats and hot flashes are a big deal. When they strike amidst the night, it's ideal to have an apparatus close by to keep fresh. Also, by "apparatus," obviously, we mean this bed fan with a remote. It's structured explicitly to scatter and keep that essential cold air legitimately between your sheets.

2. Think and concentrate far from the agony

Stress can exasperate the indications of menopause. The Mayo Clinic reports that contemplation functions as a pressure reliever, so sneak away to a private spot for a moment and practice diaphragmatic relaxing. This is when air dives deep into your midriff and not merely your mouth or lungs.

3. Go regular

Many ladies have observed essential oils to be useful for help from menopause side effects. Consider reserving a roller bottle loaded up with weakened peppermint oil by the bed for night sweats, or keeping one in your handbag for in a hurry help. A diffuser is likewise a loosening up choice to keep the room quiet and relaxed, yet don't utilize it for longer than 20 to 30 minutes like clockwork (or no longer than 1 hour at one time).

4. Switch up your eating regimen and try intermittent fasting

One study Trusted Source found that intermittent fasting (IF) can be particularly useful for weight control or weight reduction for post-menopausal ladies. There are different sorts of intermittent fasting, all which include confining your calorie consumption for a specific timespan.

Diet techniques incorporate the 5/2, 16/8, eat-stop-eat, and warrior diet. Each sort has run about how and when you eat. A few people guarantee this eating regimen improves your stomach related framework, brings down aggravation, and diminishes muscle to fat ratio. In any case, intermittent fasting can cause medical issues on the off chance that you have certain conditions, for example, diabetes or coronary illness. Converse with your specialist before trying it.

5. Grasp work out

Ladies' bodies can change all around drastically after menopause. Indeed, another study found that menopause may change how ladies' muscles use oxygen. These adjustments in the muscles imply that activity could compare to ever. As a little something extra, exercise may likewise help reduce probably the most well-known side effects, similar to weight gain, disposition changes, and weariness. For the best activities to do amid menopause, read increasingly here.

6. Analysis of toys

Hormonal changes and physical changes amid menopause can cause vaginal divider slenderness and a reduction in conventional oil. This can cause a marked decrease in charisma as well. It's essential to regard what works for your specific relationship, however on the off chance that you and your accomplice need to get things moving in the room once more, vibrators may be your answer. Studies have appeared many ladies have had accomplishment in expanding their drive and sexual fulfillment through the presentation of vibrators. There are many different kinds of vibrators available, so converse with your accomplice and analysis with one (or a few!).

Intermittent Fasting and Menopause

Intermittent fasting is a developing pattern for people. I have seen it convey astounding outcomes on my ongoing retreat and I have been animated by my companion Andy who is looking lean and stimulated in the wake of turning into an evangelist for the advantages of intermittent fasting. The benefits of intermittent fasting can include:

- More vitality
- Weight reduction
- Increment in fit bulk
- Lifts the invulnerable framework
- Insurance against certain infections because of expanded cell reestablishment
- The decrease in pressure and irritation
- Improvement of insulin affectability in overweight ladies
- Help alleviate sadness
- Lift intellectual capacity
- Strong enemy of maturing as it recovers your whole framework

Indeed, even with every one of these advantages, intermittent fasting still stays dubious the same number of individuals believe is it not protected to abandon nourishment for long periods. It has particularly being viewed as disputable for ladies as extreme eating examples can influence your periods and hormones.

Your wellbeing and ailment ought to dependably be considered, yet the truth of the matter is people have dependably fasted. Thinking back in history, you can see the fixed starting points of fasting. Mountain men would go long periods without nourishment and afterward have a banquet. It is likewise established profoundly into many societies and highlights in the book of scriptures and different religions. For many, fasting is a purifying experience.

Is intermittent fasting alright for full grown or menopausal ladies?

With so many of us effectively battling with menopause/hormone changes, hot flushes, restless evenings, and nervousness the exact opposite thing we need is an eating regimen that strengthens the indications. Every one of your hormones is interconnected, so your eating routine and eating examples can significantly impact your hormones. By fasting, you will expand the creation of the appetite hormones, ghrelin and leptin, which can make your periods progressively unpredictable (on the off chance that you are as yet having them), increment nervousness and influence rest.

Amid the menopause, ladies' bodies are increasingly touchy to any changes, so it's essential to bit by bit develop the length of the fasting window. Test it out to check whether fasting and devouring just liquids diminishes your menopause manifestations or builds them. If it expands them, it is ideal to stop as it may not be for you.

We are beginning with intermittent fasting.

Here are some prescribed procedures to help you on a smooth fasting venture:

- Begin off with a 12-hour fasting/12-hour eating window

- Step by step tries to build the fasting window from 12 to 16 hours.

- Stay away from outrageous fasting windows for more than 16 hours.

- Drink loads of solid liquids while fasting – homegrown tea, water, clear soup

- Develop your activity delicately and tune in to how your body feels

- Get some natural air – strolling, yoga, and extending all assistance, you feel the advantages.

Fitting in intermittent fasting with your life

There are many ways you can coordinate intermittent fasting into your way of life, here as some of the best ones that help the menopause:

12-16 Flexible Method

This is the most open approach to slide into intermittent fasting without annoying your hormones. You can shift your fasting window and don't need to quick consistently. You could see quick once per week or each other day.

Fasting Window: 12-16 hours/Eating Window: 8-12 hours

16/8 Method

When you need to experience a more profound intermittent experience and the advantages, at that point, try the 16/8 approach.

Fasting Window: 16 hours/Eating Window: 8 hours

5/2 and 16/8 Method

One methodology is to incorporate fasting into the well-regarded 5:2 eating routine. On the two days, seven days that you devour the 500 calories have this in an 8-hour window and quick for the remainder of the time. At that point for the other five days eat typically, with the two days with intermittent fasting.

Fasting window 16 hours for two days, typical for the rest/Eating Window: 8 hours for two days, ideal for 5

Intermittent Fasting Weight Loss (The Ultimate Weight Loss Hack)

Intermittent fasting is an eating regimen that is quickly developing in prevalence and turning into the best approach to shed pounds. A month ago alone, there were more than 246,000 looks for the expression 'intermittent fasting' on Google alone. This inquiry volume demonstrates how famous it's moved toward becoming.

Researchers and sustenance specialists like it as well and are stating it's the method for the future for losing and keeping weight off and new books on the point are being distributed daily including the smash hit books like 'Eat Stop Eat' and 'The 8 Hour Diet'. Intermittent fasting is likewise well known with supporters of the Paleo diet since our precursors seem to have eaten along these lines for a large number of years.

This part encourages all of you about intermittent fasting weight misfortune and subtleties why it is the best weight misfortune diet hack around. In the wake of understanding it, you will probably execute into your eating routine and experience the advantages it offers very quickly.

Beginning With Intermittent Fasting

Following this eating regimen plan is overly straightforward. You should pick a timeframe amid the day that you will quickly. This ought to be between 16-20 hours. The more you were quick every day, the better. Do whatever it takes not to worry over checking calories or carbohydrates. Focus on approaching your day until it's an excellent opportunity to eat.

You don't have to brisk reliably before all else either. You may be increasingly open to breaking in gradually with 2-3 fasts per week at first. Include extra-long stretches of intermittent fasting as you become increasingly alright with this style of eating.

Tips To Make Intermittent Fasting Easier

1. Amid your quick, you'll need to drink a lot of water.

Crush a little lemon or lime juice into your water to help dispose of any yearnings you experience. You can likewise drink espresso, tea, or other calorie-free refreshments. Following half a month, you will locate that intermittent fasting keeps you from wanting sugar altogether.

2. When you can deal with it, take in a little caffeine toward the beginning of the day and early evening.

The caffeine in espresso and tea may make intermittent fasting a little simpler to quick since it's useful for checking your craving. Be mindful so as not to enjoy as this may prompt you feeling a little excessively wired. I likewise prescribe these natural vitality boosting tips to keep you going amid the day.

3. Keep away from falsely seasoned beverages.

One sort of calorie-free beverage that ought to be kept away from our diet soft drinks and different refreshments that utilization artificial sugars like Splenda and Sweet and Low. Studies demonstrate that they can animate your hunger like a beverage that contains sugar and cause you to indulge.

4. Try not to glut at your first dinner.

The first feast after your quick ought to be the measure of nourishment you usually eat. Gorging will make you feel dreadful and reduce the advantages you get from the fast.

5. Minimize foods rich in prepared carbohydrates and sugars.

While intermittent fasting makes it conceivable to eat a little looser than ordinary, you should even now eat as meager bread, pasta, rice, and so forth as could be expected under the circumstances.

Focus instead on eating protein from hamburger, fish, or pork, carbohydrates from vegetables, natural product, and sweet potatoes, and solid fats from foods like almonds, avocados, fish, and olive oil.

How Intermittent Fasting Will Help You Lose Weight

Eating like this has various preferences concerning weight adversity. The first is when you're fasting, your body will be compelled to utilize its put away body fat for vitality. Consuming calories this way, rather than from the sustenance you're eating for the day, will help you get more fit as well as weight from any abundance body fat you're conveying. This implies you won't only be more slender however will likewise look preferred and be a lot more advantageous over if you get in shape as it was done in the good 'ol days.

Intermittent fasting is that it can help enhance the arrival of the critical fat consuming hormones in your body. The is particularly valid for the two most important hormones: human development hormone (HGH) and insulin.

Human development hormone assumes an essential job in turning on your bodies fat consuming heater, so it gets the calories you have to work and play from putting away body fat. Studies demonstrate that fasting can expand your body's creation of development hormone by 1,300% in ladies and 2,000% in men!

The intermittent impact fasting has on insulin is similarly as noteworthy and potentially increasingly significant. Keeping your insulin levels low and relentless is critical to losing overabundance fat and keeping it off. Diets that are rich in prepared carbohydrates (bread, pasta, rice) and straightforward sugars (sweets, treats, and soft drink) have the contrary impact. They cause your insulin levels to spike quickly and after that crash each time you eat one of these foods. The net consequence of this wonder is that your body will store a higher amount of what you eat as overabundance body fat as opposed to consuming it off as vitality.

Incessantly raising your insulin levels like this can likewise prompt the improvement of sort II diabetes, obesity, and other endless medical issues. Intermittent fasting effectively takes care of this issue.

Following an intermittent fasting style of eating regimen for 15 days is appeared in clinical examinations to help 'balance' your insulin levels. This will enable your body to remain in a calorie and fat consuming state. You'll likewise find that it gives you more vitality for the day.

Another extraordinary weight misfortune advantage of intermittent fasting is that food cravings and yearnings that may regularly torment you for the day will be diminished, if not inside and out dispensed with. This is most likely because of its capacity to adjust your insulin and glucose levels and, this way help right other hormonal uneven characters.

Intermittent Fasting Weight Loss FAQs

Since you recognize what intermittent fasting is and how to begin, it's an ideal opportunity to address your different inquiries.

The following are answers to the inquiries often posed about intermittent fasting. These answers should help you as well and make the beginning much simpler.

The amount Weight Will I Lose?

The measure of weight you lose with fasting is dictated by how frequently and long your facts are, what you eat a while later, and different elements. Fasting for 16-20 hours daily can help you securely shed 2-3 pounds of fat each week.

While losing this much weight each week is incredible, it's how it gets it going that is genuinely cool. Shedding pounds with intermittent fasting implies that you will never need to check calories or plan and set up a few dinners per day.

Would I be able to Work Out While Fasting?

Truly, you can. You are doing the right sort of exercise while fasting will enable you to get thinner quicker and even form muscle.

The best exercises to do while fasting for weight misfortune are 3-4 severe quality preparing workouts week after week. This implies anything from standard quality making to iron weight or body weight workouts.

Focus on completing 3-4 absolute body practices for every exercise with as little rest as conceivable between sets. Doing this will enable you to consume more calories amid and after your workout. You'll construct muscle too, which will allow you to look and feel better as the weight falls off.

One exercise that I've observed to be viable for weight misfortune when joined with intermittent fasting is the 10 Minute Workout plan, which should be possible at home or the rec center.

Won't I Lose Muscle When I Fast?

I wouldn't sweat this by any stretch of the imagination. Most importantly, you aren't fasting sufficiently long for your body to begin separating muscle for vitality. You have maybe a considerable number of calories from your put away body fat to use before that will start to occur. Concentrates demonstrate that even in the wake of fasting for three days, no muscle is lost.

Is Fasting Safe?

For whatever length of time that you are trustworthy, not pregnant, and aren't taking drugs, fasting is protected. Like all weight control plans, you ought to talk about it with your specialist before starting an intermittent fasting style of abstaining from excessive food intake.

I additionally feel that it may not be keen to pursue this eating routine when you're mainly pushed. Since this eating routine can be a little pressure inciting at first, doing as such when your capacity to be moderately peaceful and rested most likely is certainly not a smart thought.

Are There Any Supplements I Can Take To Make Fasting Easier?

Likewise, with some other weight misfortune plan, it's a smart thought to take a couple of dietary enhancements to guarantee that your daily necessities are met. This incorporates an on more than one occasion daily multi-nutrient, fish oil, and nutrient D.

I've likewise discovered taking 10 grams of branch chain amino acids when my workouts genuinely help as well. They're extraordinary for giving you more vitality amid your exercise and indeed diminishing post-exercise muscle soreness.

You can likewise utilize a BCAA supplement amid your quick to help lessen the danger of smashing or experiencing a terrible state of mind amid the day.

Want To Try Intermittent Fasting For Weight Loss? 7 Things You Need To Know First

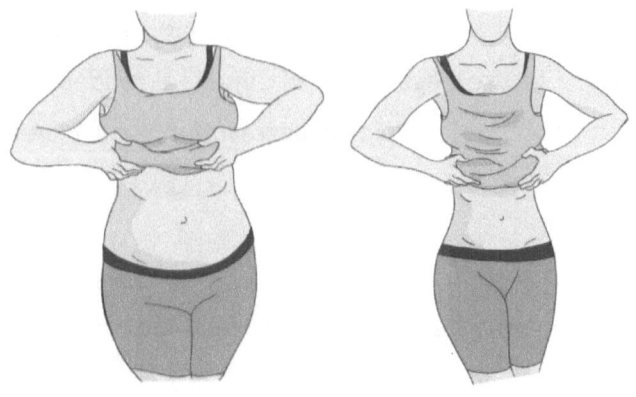

Numerous individuals have discovered weight loss success with intermittent fasting (IF). However, that doesn't mean weight loss is ensured. Here are seven things you have to know before you begin a periodic fasting program:

1. Weight loss isn't the main advantage.

Intermittent fasting has numerous medical advantages. When has been appealed to ensure against sort two diabetes by decreasing insulin obstruction; improve heart wellbeing; secure against Alzheimer's, moderate the maturing procedure; diminish aggravation, and increment mental clearness.

2. There is nobody best intermittent fasting program.

There is no "one" way or "right" approach to doing intermittent fasting. There are various strategies you can pursue. Some fasting conventions incorporate each other day fasting, two days of fasting (or outrageous calorie decrease) trailed by five days of healthy eating, 14 to 16 hours of fasting pursued by an 8-to 10-hour eating window, etc. Need to realize the best intend to pursue? The arrangement works best for you. Pick a program that works best with your timetable, your identity, and even your dietary patterns.

3. Weight loss isn't a certification.

If you figure intermittent fasting could be an incredible method to get in shape, you're correct. A few examinations, including a recent report led at the University of Illinois at Chicago, indicated intermittent fasting to be as powerful as calorie-prohibitive weight control plans. It works just whenever done accurately. That is, much the same as some other weight loss program; you have to hold fast to specific rules or standards to make it work. Following the assigned eating and fasting windows is significant, yet increasingly significant isn't overcompensating for lost calories amid one's fasting window. See beneath for additional on overcompensation.

4. Overcompensation can be a major issue.

Intermittent fasting helps weight loss since it causes you to diminish your day by day or week by week calorie utilization. When you begin overcompensating for those missed calories by devouring more nourishment all through the remainder of the day or on your non-fasting days/hours, you can undermine any desire for weight loss. If you stick to standard suppers and substantial snacks amid your eating window and don't overcompensate by overeating yourself following your quick, you have a superior possibility of having weight loss success.

5. Intermittent fasting isn't for everyone.

Specific individuals shouldn't endeavor intermittent fasting, including ladies who are pregnant or breastfeeding, youngsters or adolescents, individuals with diabetes or hypothyroidism, or who are underweight, malnourished, or have a dietary problem. Similarly, as with any new eating routine, dependably ask your human services proficient before you start.

6. It's dubious whether ladies ought to do intermittent fasting.

There is still some contention around whether intermittent fasting is directly for ladies because of the danger of hormone lopsidedness. Even though reviews on rodents have indicated hormone lopsidedness and even fruitlessness, the jury is still out on the risks for ladies. Until the progressively solid proof is accessible, it might be best, to begin with, an intermittent fasting plan that is less outrageous. For instance, ladies should go for a 13-to 14-hour fasting window as opposed to a 15-to 16-hour window or a throughout the day quick. When you are holding fast to a program that calls for calorie restriction on many days, is brilliant and doesn't confine your calories to an extraordinary dimension or for back to back days.

7. Intermittent fasting isn't an eating regimen.

Intermittent fasting is a calendar, not an eating routine. A healthy eating routine states what you can and can't eat. Intermittent fasting doesn't confine any nourishments yet instead gives a timetable or example to eating with windows of eating or fasting.

Eat Stop Eat Review - Intermittent Fasting For Weight Loss

Some information on Eat Stop Eat:

Weight loss has dependably been an issue, in any event since society pronounced that thin individuals are delightful and that individuals begin to get worried about wellbeing perils like cholesterol, diabetes obesity, etc. Thus, one of the undeniably popular weight loss techniques is, obviously the quick strategy. There's a popular choice these days, an ongoing achievement on the weight loss specialty called Eat Stop Eat.

Wellbeing and Weight:

Wellbeing is exceptionally corresponded with your weight, since being overweight methods you are bringing about significantly more wellbeing dangers than if you have a healthy pressure, in that capacity, Eat Stop Eat can enable you to get more benefits in a viable manner.

Exercise, what amount, and when?

The program will reveal to you precisely the amount you need to practice and exactly when to exercise to have the best outcomes - maxing the calorie consume and improving your endeavors.

Longer Fasts versus Intermittent Fasts:

There is sufficient logical data at this point to safely express that more drawn out fasts are risky for one's wellbeing, and that intermittent fasts, similarly as in the Eat Stop Eat diet, have no threats and are the most exhorted arrangement, so you can make sure you won't get any wellbeing dangers while on the program - an incredible opposite.

Keep Muscle Mass and Energy Levels High:

One significant concern individuals have with regards to Fasts is that they will most likely lose their bulk and get that endless exhaustion settled in. With this eating routine, you won't need to stress over that, as you will keep that well-deserved bulk and your vitality levels will be held high consistently, even on your "quick occasions."

Controlling your Metabolism:

Controlling your digestion or giving your digestion a chance to control you is the thing that settles the contrast among this and other fasting programs. When you quick you, for the most part, feels the distinction and reacts by bringing down your digestion speed and entering survival mode, implying that it will attempt to keep each since calorie you give it. With Eat Stop Eat you won't get your endeavors ruined by your digestion, you won't enter "survival mode" so you will lose calories quicker than with some other pill out there.

Along these lines, summing up, Eat Stop Eat is a technique that truly brings a different age upon the weight loss specialty and reforms how we quick - so make a point to consider this strategy if you need to lose those additional pounds.

CONCLUSION

Safe fasting for weight reduction is the way to effectively consuming muscle to fat ratio with intermittent fasting. The issue anyway is that numerous individuals plunge into utilizing fasting to get more fit without realizing how to do as such safely. What happens is they end up inclination weary and put their health in danger. Fortunately, it shouldn't be like this, and fasting can be a powerful and safe approach to weight reduction.

Right off the bat, we ought to elucidate what fasting is and what it isn't. Fasting is a drawn-out time of restraint from sustenance amid which water might be smashed, and a few people likewise have juice fasts in which they can drink different sorts of juice. Intermittent fasting involves alternating periods of fasting, with periods of eating with the general mean to confine calorie utilization and accomplish a calorie shortfall.

One precedent is exchange day sustaining where a 24 hour quick is trailed by multi-day where sustenance might be expended; another path is to take into consideration a little three to four-hour eating window eventually amid the day. Both of these strategies are safe and have been appeared to have positive health benefits notwithstanding weight reduction, for example, bringing down of glucose levels.

The risky emerge when individuals attempt outrageous fasts for a couple of days or more, definitely decreasing nourishment admission like this will abandon you feeling worn out, sleepy, woozy and wiped out. Consequently, safe fasting for weight reduction ought to involve short periods of fasting pursued by periods of reasonable, healthy, moderate sustenance utilization.